The TRAIN HAPPY *Journal*

30 DAYS TO KICK START YOUR INTUITIVE MOVEMENT JOURNEY

TALLY RYE

PAVILION

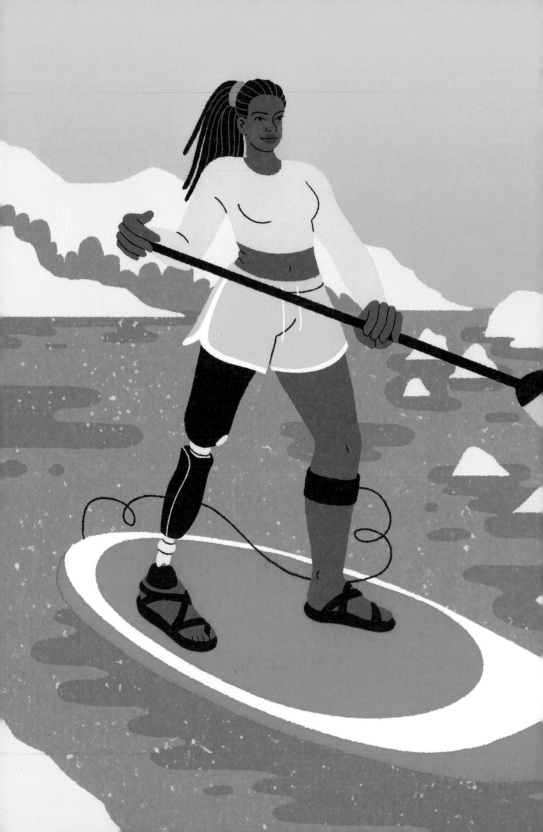

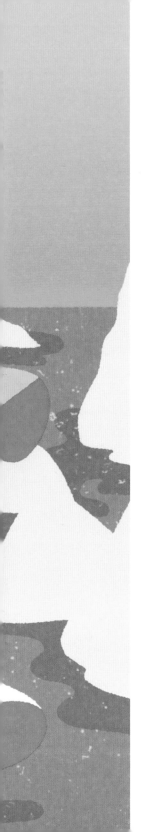

CONTENTS

INTRODUCTION

Welcome to the *Train Happy Journal*, the counterpart to my book *Train Happy*. In a nutshell, the Train Happy ethos is about helping you to build a happy and healthy relationship with movement. Exercise is no longer about punishing your body. Instead, exercise is about working with your body, so it can become an important form of self-care. I hope this journal will deepen your understanding of the Train Happy ethos and that the daily tasks help to bring the principles of intuitive movement to life so you can apply them to your own fitness journey.

The goal of intuitive movement is to create more trust and connection with your body so that you are both back on the same team. In contrast, diet culture (the messaging centred around the belief that in order to be happy, successful, fit, healthy and attractive, you must be slim) has long pitted us against our bodies, gaslighting us into believing that we cannot be trusted to make the best decisions for our health, fitness and wellbeing. It's why we blame and berate ourselves for not living up to the body ideals celebrated by diet culture: 'I could have the dream body if only I was more dedicated! If only I had more will power!' It's why we find ourselves stuck in the diet cycle, resenting fitness and resenting our bodies. But the truth is, you aren't the problem, diet culture is. (You can read more about this in *Train Happy*.)

And so the aim of this journal is to help you be proactive in rebuilding trust in your own judgement. It offers a new perspective on what fitness can be for you by challenging your beliefs about exercise and your body, so that you can have the happy and healthy relationship with movement that you deserve. In *Train Happy*, I wrote about how rebuilding this relationship can often be like untangling a necklace; slowly loosening one little bit at a time can help to gently unravel the chain so it becomes something we love and want to wear again. This is exactly what I hope the intuitive movement framework and the activities in this journal can be for you – an opportunity to gently assess and loosen the areas of your relationship with movement that may be twisted and muddled, so that you are able to see clearly how you can enjoy exercise on your terms and make fitness fun again.

So, before you dig in to the 30-Day Challenge, let's remind ourselves of the principles of intuitive movement and how they can be used as helpful signposts as you start down this new path.

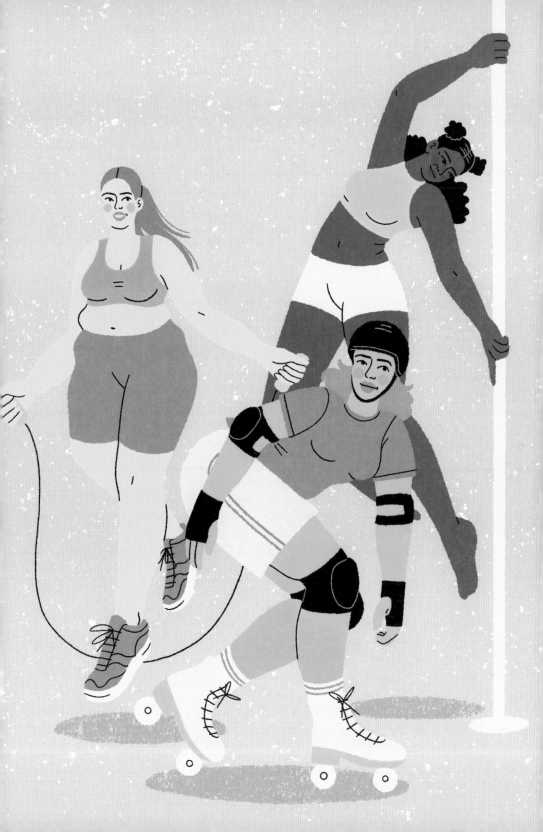

9 PRINCIPLES OF INTUITIVE MOVEMENT

Let's start with a refresher on the principles of intuitive movement. These principles have been inspired by and adapted from the 10 principles of intuitive eating, which were originally created by two dietitians, Evelyn Tribole and Elyse Resch. I felt that in the same way intuitive eating zooms in on and examines our relationship with food, we needed to hold the magnifying glass up to our relationship with exercise, because for many, that relationship can be just as fraught and unhappy.

The 9 principles of intuitive movement were created so we could ask ourselves some important questions about how we feel about moving our bodies and why we approach exercise in the way that we do.

Each principle is not a rule and this is not a step-by-step process. Instead, I encourage you to use these principles to guide you, to help you to reconnect with your body, and to trust your inner wisdom as you learn to find the fun and joy in movement again.

1. Reject the Diet Mentality
2. Honour Your Appetite for Movement
3. Unconditional Permission to Rest (stop when satisfied)
4. Make Peace with Exercise
5. Challenge the Fitness Police
6. Discover the Feel-Good Factor
7. Manage Emotions
8. Accept Your Body
9. Gentle Guidance

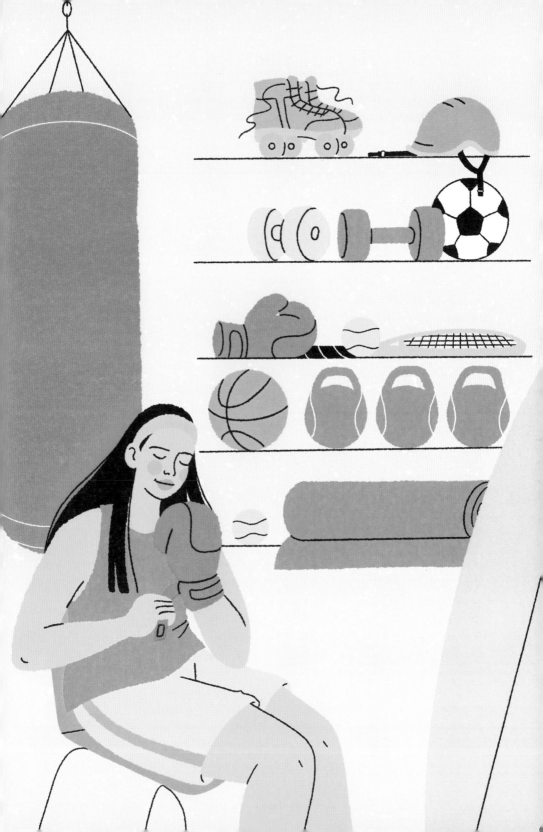

1. REJECT THE DIET MENTALITY

Diet culture taught us that exercise was just a means to an end for weight loss and aesthetic manipulation. It wasn't fun anymore. What was once playtime as a young child became something we felt obligated to do. A form of punishment to endure to compensate for other aspects of our lifestyle (like eating and drinking) so that ultimately we could conform to society's body and beauty standards. But we want it to be playtime again! Because moving your body can and should be an opportunity for adults to let loose and play.

Rejecting the diet mentality requires you to shelve the idea that the purpose of regular exercise is to achieve an intentional weight-loss or aesthetic goal. Instead, you must make (and continue to make) the choice to shift the intention behind how you choose to move. We can enjoy the wonderful benefits of regular movement without weight loss and changes to our aesthetic appearance having to be the focus and necessary outcome. (See my book *Train Happy* for more on this.)

So where do we start? By unlearning the narratives diet culture created about exercise and choosing to try a different approach.

A) RECOGNIZE & ACKNOWLEDGE THE HARM DIETS DO

Using exercise as a tool to control our weight is not only largely unsustainable, it can also negatively impact our mental health. For many, this can include physical discomfort from punishing workouts, feelings of guilt and shame about food and body, anxiety when taking rest, and fear of not meeting society's beauty and body standards. How has diet culture impacted your relationship with fitness? Has it made it more complicated and stressful? By focusing on weight and aesthetics, have you been stuck in a cycle of feeling like your body is never good enough? This is something we will address later on in the journal.

B) BE AWARE OF THE DIET MENTALITY TRAITS & MINDSET

Our view of fitness is largely shaped by snippets of fitness content and diet tips we have absorbed over the years. From books, websites, magazines, podcasts, TV shows... we have consciously and subconsciously picked up so much information that reinforces the idea that exercise

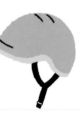

is for burning calories and 'sculpting' your body only. As we start to become aware of the stories we tell ourselves about fitness, it's important we reflect on where these narratives have come from and how they have made an impact on us and our relationship with exercise. By increasing our awareness of where our diet tips and tricks have come from, we can begin to bust the myths and start the healing process.

C) GET RID OF THE DIET TOOLS

What tools are you using which reinforce the diet culture agenda that exercise is about earning and burning food to achieve your dream body? Perhaps it's your fitness watch, an app on your phone, a diet book on your shelf or the scales in your bathroom. We will work on getting rid of the tools that no longer serve you, and setting boundaries so you have the space to heal.

D) BE KIND AND COMPASSIONATE TO YOURSELF

Unlearning years, maybe decades, of diet culture is tough. Please cut yourself some slack as you start swimming against the tide. Once you take off the rose-tinted glasses, you will see how much diet culture has not only negatively impacted you but the people around you. There may be times when you feel angry and frustrated about the time spent trying to achieve the unrealistic standards set. You may also miss the coping mechanisms diet culture taught you to use as you learn to build new self-care tools. Moving away from diet culture is like leaving a toxic relationship and, though you know it's for the best, there is likely to be a sense of grief as part of you misses the familiarity. It will feel challenging, and it's likely you'll want to go back at times. So, know that that is to be expected and show the compassion and kindness you would give to others to yourself.

When working through this journal and the 30-Day Challenge, you may feel overwhelmed at times. The key thing with any intuitive movement journey is to **go at your own pace**. We want to make you the expert of your body again. So remember that these principles, and this journal, are here to guide you, but ultimately you can do this inner work in your own time.

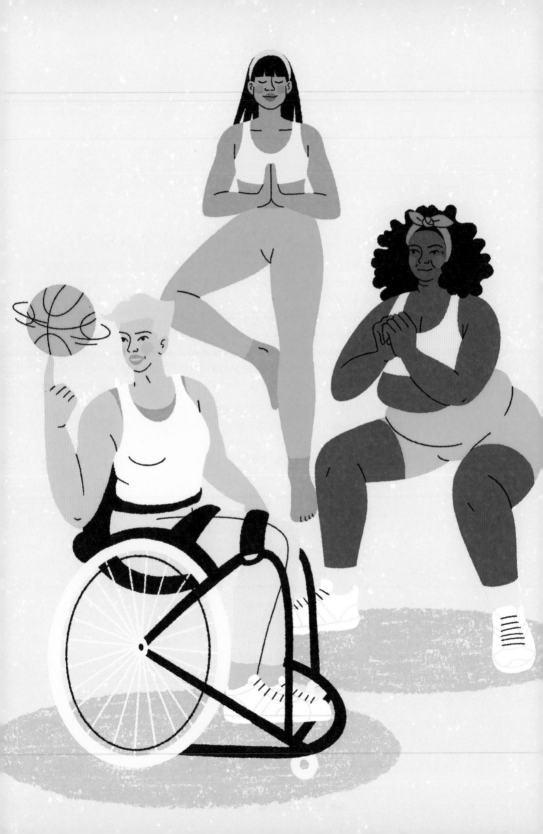

2. HONOUR YOUR APPETITE FOR MOVEMENT

Do you know what kind of workouts you actually like? Or have you been doing what you 'should' be doing because you read that a particular type of workout was best for fat burn? I love to ask this question: If exercise had zero impact on your weight or appearance, how would you choose to move?

So many of us are disconnected from our preferences when it comes to movement and have never considered them before. How do you like to move? What time of day feels best? Where is your favourite place to be active? These are just a few of the questions you will be working through as you learn what works for you. Because funnily enough, what's best for you and your lifestyle is likely to be very different to the recommendation that a PT gave you in a one-off consultation after knowing you for five minutes.

Use this principle as a way to get curious about movement and to try different things before you figure out what works for you. Honouring your movement appetite helps you to continue building trust and strengthen the connection with your body through interoceptive awareness (the process in which your brain receives, understands and responds to information about the physical sensations within your body).

3. UNCONDITIONAL PERMISSION TO REST (STOP WHEN SATISFIED)

The principles of intuitive movement are not just about helping you to reframe exercise; they are about helping you to reframe rest too. Rest is just as beneficial and as important as movement can be for the body, but so many of us fear it may 'undo all our hard work'. But what does that mean? Where did that fear come from? And why would it be so catastrophic for our hard work to be undone? I'm sure we can trace those breadcrumbs back to diet culture once again.

Rest may also feel like you're relinquishing control, and that will be the case for some. Rigid exercise can be used as a means to control our body and our emotions. Resting and just 'being' is challenging in a world that validates hustle, productivity and grind. Learning to just 'be' is an essential part of the healing process, not just for our bodies but for our minds too. And so, by opening up to the idea of rest, we become open to giving space and time to the inner work that we may have been literally and figuratively running away from. Taking a break from formal movement may be a necessary endeavour as you learn to reorientate your relationship with movement (see pages 20–21).

On a physical level, rest is about giving your body an opportunity to process the training stimulus and make the adaptations it needs to come back stronger. However, to make peace with rest we must give ourselves unconditional permission to rest our body at *all times*. That may mean stopping during a workout if you need to, taking a day to recover or perhaps even a week, month or more. Knowing that you are always entitled to leave the class, stop mid-activity, or stay at home, can give you and your body the assurance that if and when it gives you the signals and cues for rest, you will honour that. And once again, honouring your body's needs will continue to strengthen your relationship with it. If you feel unsure, anxious and conflicted about rest, then the activities in this journal are designed to help rest become an important and celebrated act of self-care.

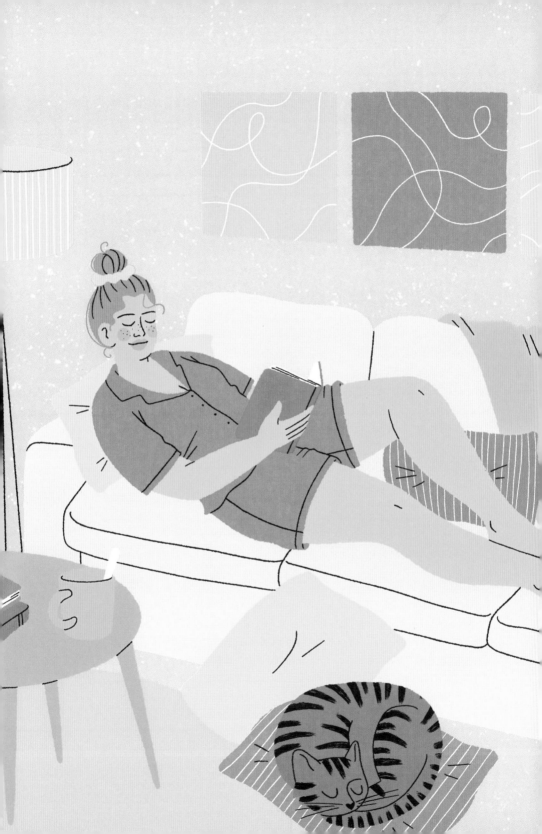

4. MAKE PEACE WITH EXERCISE

What has your relationship with exercise been in the past? Perhaps the word exercise itself brings on feelings of restriction and forced workouts? It's why I like to talk about movement, physical activity and fitness, as it helps to broaden our view of what 'exercise' is, because it extends far beyond your PE classes at school and the four walls of a gym.

This principle is partly about reflecting on your movement history and how it has moulded your view of fitness and physical activity. You may have dreaded exercise after having a traumatic PE experience, or become obsessed with it after a positive one, never missing a workout. You may have only used exercise as a dieting tool, going along with whatever workout your diet said was effective, and have never explored what you actually enjoy doing? Or maybe a different scenario entirely?

Diet culture has undeniably had an impact on the way we view fitness. One way it has done this is by making us categorize certain types of exercise as 'good' and others as 'bad'. Often the 'good' exercise would be the one deemed to be the most efficient for calorie burn and aesthetic results. The 'bad' exercise may be considered a waste of time because it supposedly didn't achieve the aesthetic results you were after, didn't make you sweat enough or (your fitness watch said) didn't raise your heart rate enough.

Making peace with exercise is about letting go of this binary view, and recognizing that all movement is valid, and that there are so many wonderful ways to move your body. **All movement counts.** Ultimately, the best workout is the one you *enjoy* and therefore can do consistently – this principle also helps us to find enjoyment in movement again by encouraging us to let go of the narrow way diet culture views fitness.

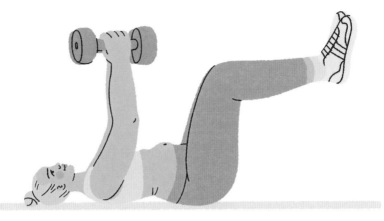

5. CHALLENGE THE FITNESS POLICE

Diet culture gave us a lot of rules about exercise and with them a lot of guilt, anxiety and shame about sticking (or not sticking) to those rules in the process. Some may be as obvious as 'never miss a Monday', or as subtle as 'I must always be sore the next day or it doesn't count'. In fact, the idea of whether certain types of exercise 'count' or are seen as valid is often a significant part of how we view fitness, so this is where we challenge that. Who made the rules? Where did they come from? What happens when I break the rules?

Well, as we know, rules are made to be broken, and in this case it's no different. This principle is about reflecting on the rules and restrictions you may have experienced, so you can challenge them, overcome them and rebuild trust in yourself. In the 30-Day Challenge we will examine and identify the rules you have followed, rebel against those rules and reflect on how we feel about that process. It may be the case that you need to keep challenging the same rules several times for you to overcome the fear created by diet culture. But each time you do challenge them, the diet culture voice gets weaker and your inner voice becomes more powerful.

6. DISCOVER THE FEEL-GOOD FACTOR

Moving your body should be something that makes you feel better about yourself, not worse. For so long exercise has been seen as either a punishment, a chore that should be endured, or something we feel obligated to do so we can keep up with body and beauty standards. But it can be so much more than that. It can and should be a wonderful form of self-care. That's not to say that it's always sunshine and rainbows – sometimes it's really challenging and difficult in the moment. But, that discomfort should feel worth it, as it supports your physical and mental wellbeing, building your confidence and self-esteem in the process.

Feeling good for you may mean more than the release of endorphins. It may mean finding and growing a sense of pride, confidence, social connection, self-celebration, inner strength and resilience. Figuring out not only the right type of movement for you, but how it positively impacts you, is also a vital part of building a deeper motivation. By understanding how regular movement contributes to how you feel physically and mentally, we can start to create a list of reasons, intrinsic to you, that make you want to keep coming back to the activities which give you that spark.

Throughout the 30-Day Challenge we will explore how the workouts you enjoy make you feel.

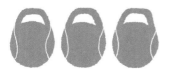

7. MANAGE EMOTIONS

Exercise is often considered to be a helpful therapy. You may have heard fitness professionals regularly tout exercise as a cure-all for mental health. However, this is unhelpful and misleading, as while exercise is certainly therapeutic and can massively help us to cope with our emotions as part of a larger self-care toolkit, it does not directly address the deeper issues and emotions we may need to deal with. It should never be solely relied upon as a way to address our mental health.

Sadly, because many do over-rely on exercise to help deal with their mental health, it can lead to an obsessive and unhealthy relationship with exercise as a means to control and distract from the deeper wounds inside that may need healing. As mentioned in principle 3, rest may actually be a huge part of how you learn to give space to, and understand, your emotions. Slowing down physically, so you have time and energy to explore other forms of emotional support, can be extremely beneficial for your mental wellbeing as well as your relationship with movement.

And when we have a positive relationship with movement that is founded on self-care, we can then learn to use movement as a helpful way to soothe and connect us with our emotions.

Moving our bodies may be a crucial way in which we complete the stress cycle and manage the physical aspect of our mental health. They're not called 'feelings' for nothing – they are designed to be felt physically. Which is why we feel anxiety in our chest, and nerves in our tummy. And so, emotion = energy in motion. It has to have somewhere to go. So rather than using exercise as a way to numb our feelings, we can use it to connect us to them. Therefore, when we do have more self-care tools in our kit, movement may become an important one for you but no longer the only one.

8. ACCEPT YOUR BODY

Historically, we know that exercise has been pitched as a tool to manipulate our aesthetic, and so working out became the way to achieve that dream body for so many. Me very much included. We've been fighting our bodies through exercise to fit body and beauty standards in the same way we try to bash a square peg into a round hole. We have blamed and berated our appearance for not being good enough or worthy enough. But really it was diet culture and its fat-phobic beauty standards that failed us.

Unlearning this story we have been telling ourselves for so long takes time, inner strength (that I know you have) and compassion. Accepting your body is not an overnight thing. We can't snap our fingers and make it happen. However, finding joy in movement, and building your confidence through **celebrating who you are and what your body can do** instead of what it looks like, can be a key part of writing a new narrative.

The myth that fitness has a 'look' and is only for people who fit that narrow ideal, meant that for so long the fitness industry and its clientele have felt like an exclusive club. And if you didn't fit that mould, then the only reason you would be there is to change your body into one that did.

But no more. Fitness is for everyone and every body. Fit bodies come in all shapes and sizes and you don't need to wait on your weight to start your own fitness journey today.

The challenges in this journal are designed to help build your self-esteem and confidence, so not only do you realize (and internalize) that you are more than your appearance and your body, but that you have so many great things to offer this world. What would happen if you were able to let go and show up exactly as you wanted to?

9. GENTLE GUIDANCE

The final piece in the puzzle and, as I like to think of it, the cherry on the cake. As you work through the other aspects of your relationship with fitness, we use principle 9 to start reintroducing structure, goal setting and guidance. It may take you a while to get to this point, but the aim is to be able to work towards your fitness goals with flexibility instead of fear.

The rest of the framework is to help you work on the intention behind your workouts, but gentle guidance helps you to approach *what* you are doing in an intuitive movement way. There is a common misconception that intuitive movers just train randomly and sporadically and don't focus on specific goals. While there may be a period where you don't have much structure and routine and go with how you feel, that won't always be an appropriate way to approach a fitness goal and some structure will need to be introduced.

You will know you are ready to incorporate this principle when you are no longer operating from a place of fear, but out of curiosity and excitement to build and improve your own physical performance. Perhaps you may want to work towards a new running PB, swim a new distance or learn to do your first pull-up? Improving physical performance, rather than manipulating your appearance, can be hugely encouraging as you embark on your fitness journey long term. Incorporating flexibility – including opportunity to rest, reschedule and allow room for manoeuvre – in our training plans, means that we move away from the rigidity that diet culture touted as the only way. Instead, we move towards a more sustainable approach to fitness that no longer bypasses you, and instead honours you, your body and its needs.

We will look more closely into the specifics of how to track your fitness progress and incorporate gentle guidance towards the end of the 30-Day Challenge (see pages 88–91). However, this may be something you come back to later, as only you know when the timing is right.

THE INTUITIVE MOVEMENT JOURNEY

The aim of this journal is to help kick-start your journey away from the diet mentality so that you can work towards finding your Intuitive Movement Sweet Spot (see the Intuitive Movement Pendulum opposite). As I have said, there is not a set timeline for this journey and it's very likely to go beyond the 30-Day Challenge in this journal.

It's also important to reiterate the principles themselves are not a step-by-step process. You may actually find you are working on certain aspects simultaneously and that different principles overlap as you focus on the various parts of your relationship with movement.

Every person who uses this journal will have had different experiences with fitness, diet culture and their body, so please never compare yourself to anyone else. Instead, focus on taking the small steps that build up to create a big shift not only in how you think and feel about exercise, but in how you think and feel about yourself.

Depending on your experience in the Diet Mentality Phase, you may need the pendulum to swing hard in the opposite direction to the F*** It Phase, as you unlearn and rebel against everything you have been taught about fitness. And it may need to stay there some time before you find a new middle ground where you and your relationship with movement can thrive.

You will find that sweet spot, whether it takes 30 days, 3 months or 3 years. And I hope that all the tasks in this journal will be helpful in the initial 30 days and far beyond. Keep coming back to them and revisiting them as old thoughts reoccur and new challenges arise.

INTUITIVE MOVEMENT PENDULUM

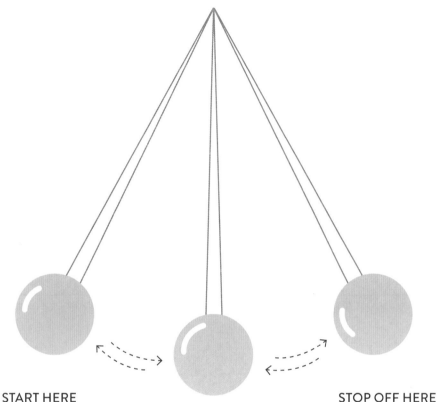

START HERE

FINAL DESTINATION

STOP OFF HERE

DIET MENTALITY PHASE

- Restriction
- Guilt & shame
- All-or-nothing approach
- Rigid mindset
- 'Should' work out
- Only weight/aesthetic-based goals

INTUITIVE MOVEMENT SWEET SPOT

- Movement is self-care
- Rest without guilt
- Fitness is a feeling not a look
- Joyful movement
- Listen to the body
- Performance-based fitness goals
- Flexible structure/routine

F*** IT PHASE

- Little/no movement
- Reject diet mentality
- Rebel against old rules
- No structure
- Rest to recover

HOW THE JOURNAL WILL WORK

The 30-Day Challenge I have created for this journal has been designed so that you can bring intuitive movement to life and feel confident in knowing how to apply the 9 principles to your own relationship with movement.

There is one challenge per day; however, you may well choose to do the tasks at your own pace and take your time, coming back to the journal when you're ready. If there are sticking points within the journal, or things you struggle with, I encourage you to revisit and repeat them at the right time for you. You may also find that you need more room to write your answers and expand on the activities, so you'll find extra note pages for you to use scattered throughout the challenge pages and on pages 104–110.

I want to emphasize that each intuitive movement journey is unique and there is no one set path. Some things that may feel fairly straightforward for you, may be a real challenge for someone else. I am not the expert of you, and neither is anybody else. The next 30 days and beyond are about helping you to reclaim and rediscover your inner dialogue so that you feel more confident and assured when making choices about your own physical and mental health and fitness.

The path may not be straightforward and sometimes you might feel like you're taking two steps back to take one step forward. But remain curious and compassionate with yourself throughout. All of these moments are opportunities to learn. Throughout the journal, you'll find real-life 'Train Happy Moments' (see page 95) to inspire and remind you to keep looking for the joy in movement and celebrate your wins against diet culture.

There is no such thing as a perfect intuitive mover and there isn't a wrong or right way to do this, so embrace the discomfort of trying something new and figure it out as you go.

MY BODY IS AN INSTRUMENT TO BE USED, NOT AN ORNAMENT TO BE LOOKED AT

Beauty Redefined

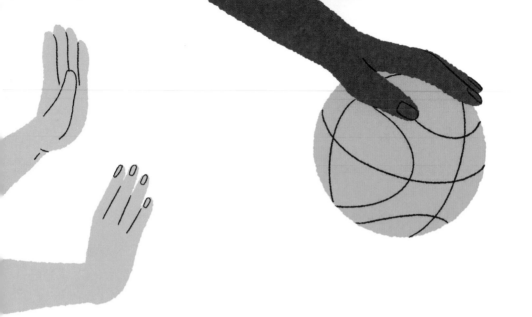

30-DAY
CHALLENGE

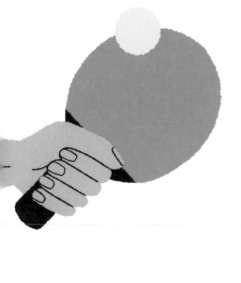

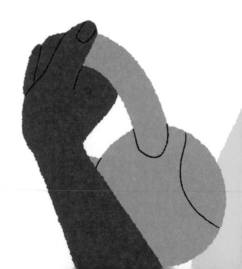

MY INTUITIVE MOVEMENT MOOD METER

Circle the numbers below to reflect how you currently feel about movement.

How do you feel about movement?

| 0 | 1 | 2 | (3) | 4 | 5 | 6 | 7 | 8 | 9 | 10 |

🙁   😐   🙂

How motivated to move do you feel?

| 0 | 1 | 2 | (3) | 4 | 5 | 6 | 7 | 8 | 9 | 10 |

🙁   😐   🙂

How do you feel about your body image?

| 0 | 1 | (2) | 3 | 4 | 5 | 6 | 7 | 8 | 9 | 10 |

🙁   😐   🙂

How do you feel about your mental wellbeing?

| 0 | 1 | 2 | 3 | 4 | 5 | 6 | (7) | 8 | 9 | 10 |

🙁   😐   🙂

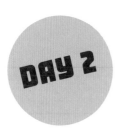

DAY 2

TAKE A BREAK FROM TRACKING MOVEMENT

Do you use a fitness watch, app or tech to track your workouts, steps or heart rate? A key part of embracing intuitive movement is to reject the diet mentality and get rid of dieting tools whilst working on your relationship with movement.

It's important that for the next 30 days you are able to take a break from your fitness tracker and apps. If this feels too hard, try taking your fitness tracker off for a day and reflect on how it feels. Then slowly build the time up from there to another day, and another, and gradually you will build up to weeks.

WHY do you track your movement?

_____

_____

_____

_____

_____

_____

How would it feel to take a break from tracking?

_____

_____

_____

_____

_____

_____

Come back and fill these in as we work through the 30-Day Challenge.
How did it feel to take a break from tracking...

After 1 day:

_____

_____

_____

_____

_____

_____

After 1 week:

_____

_____

_____

_____

_____

After 30 days:

_____

_____

_____

_____

_____

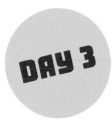

DAY 3

WORKOUT RULES

Here we reflect on the workout rules you have and where you first learnt these rules.

What workout rules do you have?	Where do they come from?
Example: I have to burn a certain number of calories before I'm allowed to stop.	*Example: Fitness account on social media.*

We'll revisit workout rules later on in the journal. (See pages 48, 64 and 84.)

"

Before my Train Happy journey I had strict mental 'rules' about what was considered acceptable and unacceptable movement. Much of the movement that I now enjoy didn't used to 'count' when I was caught up in diet culture.

– KRISTA

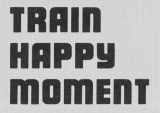

TRAIN
HAPPY
MOMENT

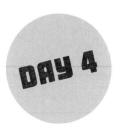

DAY 4

LEARNING TO LISTEN TO YOUR BODY

HOW DOES IT FEEL WHEN YOUR BODY ASKS FOR REST?

Draw around/on the body the feelings and sensations you experience. For example: *low energy, shaky, sore...*

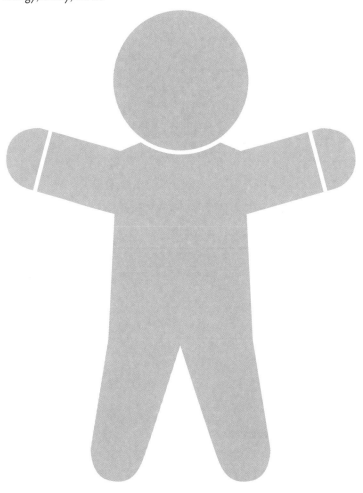

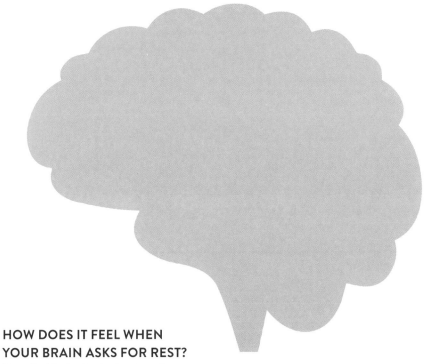

HOW DOES IT FEEL WHEN YOUR BRAIN ASKS FOR REST?

Draw inside the brain the thoughts and sensations you feel. For example: *foggy, thinking about food...*

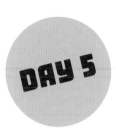

DAY 5

BUILD YOUR IDEAL REST DAY

Diet culture has taught us to fear rest days, so we are going to reframe rest days as a self-care practice.

Complete the sentences below to create your ideal rest day.

I wake up at... _____

I spend my morning... _____

_____

I make my favourite lunch of... _____

_____

In the afternoon I do... _____

_____

In the evening I have my favourite meal... _____

_____

At the end of the day, I reflect on 3 things I feel grateful for...

1. _____

2. _____

3. _____

What else would you like to include in your ideal rest day?

_____

_____

_____

"

I learnt that once I tune out diet culture I can enjoy my workout!

– CHRISTAL

TRAIN HAPPY MOMENT

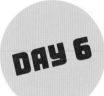

DAY 6

GETTING TO KNOW YOU

We're shifting the focus from worrying about what you look like, to celebrating **WHO** you are.

What 5 words would you use to describe yourself?

1. _____

2. _____

3. _____

4. _____

5. _____

What 5 words would your loved ones use to describe you?

1. _____

2. _____

3. _____

4. _____

5. _____

What 3 things are you most proud of?

1. _____
   _____
   _____

2. _____
   _____
   _____

3. _____
   _____
   _____

How easy was it to answer these questions about yourself?

| 0 | 1 | 2 | 3 | 4 | 5 | 6 | 7 | 8 | 9 | 10 |

Hard   Okay   Very Easy

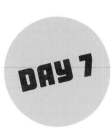

DAY 7

BUILDING MY SELF-CARE PRACTICES

Remember, exercise can be therapeutic, but it's not a replacement for therapy.

It's time to expand your self-care toolkit. In what other ways can you care for your mental wellbeing alongside movement?

In the self-care bubble below I have added some ideas, but please add more of your own.

As we work through this 30-Day Challenge and beyond, add in new self-care practices that work for you in the bubble opposite.

SELF-CARE BUBBLE

ART

JOURNAL

SOCIAL PLANS

COOK

SING

CALL A FRIEND OR LOVED ONE

BREATH WORK

SLEEP ROUTINE

MINDFUL ACTIVITIES

BUILD YOUR OWN BUBBLE

Add a new self-care practice to the bubble each week!

Take time to pamper! (Bath, feet, facepack) etc.

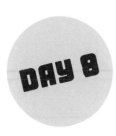

DAY 8

WORKING WITH YOUR BODY, NOT AGAINST IT

Intuitive movement is about reconnecting with your body so that you're finally back on the same team again.

Use the table below to reflect on how you may respond differently to each scenario, based on whether you are in the mindset of working with your body (even if you're not there yet) or against it.

SCENARIO	When I work with my body	When I work against my body
Alarm set for 7am workout but I had a really bad night's sleep		
I had a big celebratory meal and drinks with friends at the weekend		
My workout top is a little snug		
I feel a little under the weather		

What were the main differences for you?

_____

_____

_____

_____

_____

_____

_____

_____

_____

What surprised you about these two different approaches?

_____

_____

_____

_____

_____

_____

_____

_____

_____

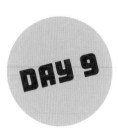

ALL MOVEMENT COUNTS

There are so many wonderful ways to move our bodies beyond those confined to the gym! This challenge is designed to expand your workout horizons, help you get curious and find more ways to be active that you enjoy.

YOGA

ICE SKATING

BARRE

POWERLIFTING

PILATES

CLIMBING

ROLLER SKATING

MARTIAL ARTS

SWIMMING

RUGBY

CYCLING

TRAMPOLINING

HIKING

DANCING

SURFING

FOOTBALL

Add more ways to move in this box:

Make a list of 10 ways to move that you are curious to try:

1. _____   6. _____

2. _____   7. _____

3. _____   8. _____

4. _____   9. _____

5. _____   10. _____

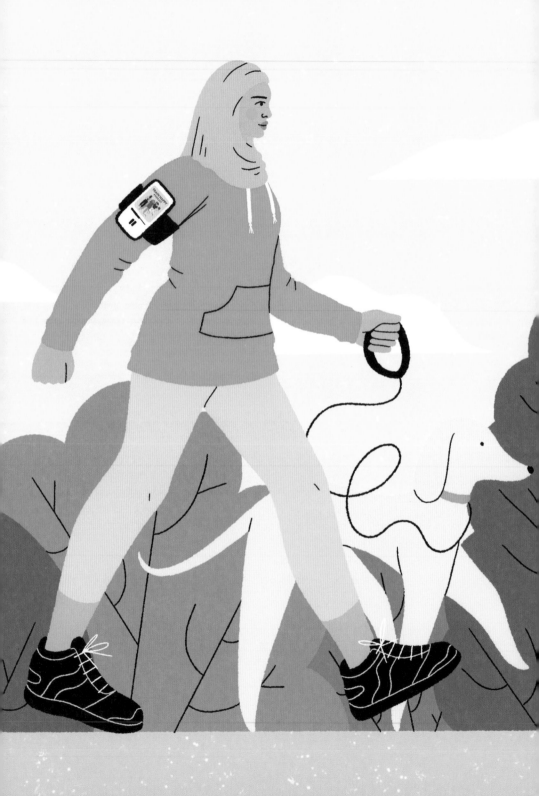

"

I've allowed myself to take walking breaks during my run without judging myself. I'm also taking child's pose breaks whenever my body asks for one during yoga class. Listening to my body while I build strength has allowed me to find so much joy in movement!

– REBECCA K

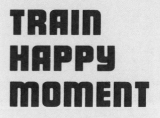

TRAIN
HAPPY
MOMENT

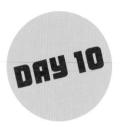

DAY 10

CLEANSE YOUR SOCIAL MEDIA FEED

ASK YOURSELF THESE QUESTIONS ABOUT THE PEOPLE YOU FOLLOW. IF YOU ANSWER 'YES' THIS IS A RED FLAG TO UNFOLLOW OR MUTE!

When you go on their page, do you compare yourself (and your body) to them?

Do they say or imply that if you eat/exercise the way they do then you could look like them?

Do they post before and after transformations and always praise a smaller body?

Do they use diet culture language to promote their workouts? E.g. 'lean', 'shred, 'fat burn', 'small waist' etc.

Are their images often heavily filtered and photoshopped?

Do they speak badly about and/or shame people with larger bodies?

Write down 3 social media accounts that make you feel good, and why.

1. _____

_____

2. _____

_____

3. _____

_____

"

I'm in the early stages of my Train Happy journey but I can already see how it's changing the way I feel about and see myself. By being able to recognize the difference between health and diet culture, I have found a new sense of pride in my body and what it can do rather than what it looks like.

– NICOLA

TRAIN HAPPY MOMENT

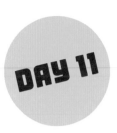

DECONSTRUCTING YOUR WORKOUT RULES

Choose one of your workout rules from Day 3 (see page 30) and deconstruct it by answering these questions.

What's the rule?

_____

_____

Where did the rule come from?

_____

_____

How do you feel if you don't stick to this rule?

_____

_____

_____

_____

_____

How could you challenge this rule and break it in the future?

_____

_____

_____

_____

_____

Notes

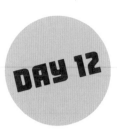

YOUR WEIGHT DOES NOT EQUAL YOUR WORTH

Create your own mantras to repeat to yourself in the mirror during your workout or when you feel challenged by diet culture.

You may also like to write these down on a sticky note and put them on your mirror for a morning reminder.

I am proud that I'm a _____ , _____ , _____ person.

My body is amazing because...

_____

_____

I am strong because...

_____

_____

I choose to celebrate my...

_____

_____

The best thing about my personality is...

_____

_____

_____

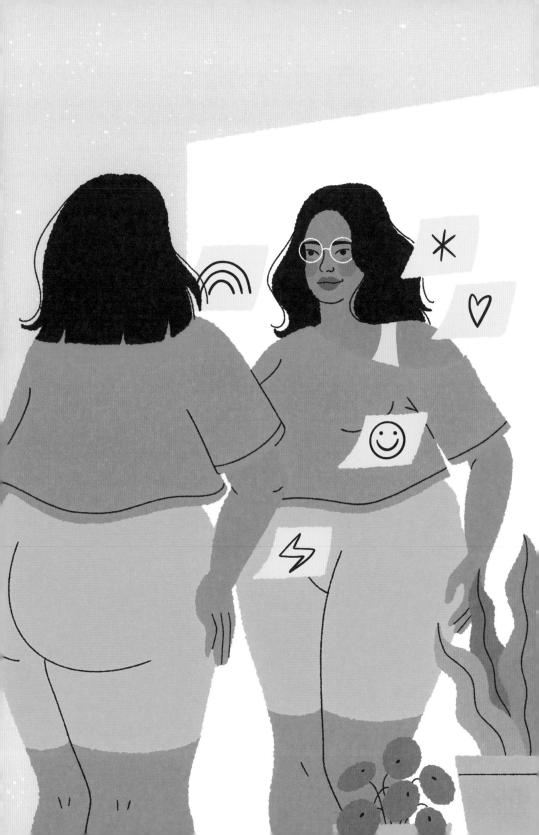

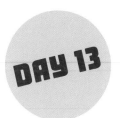

GETTING TO KNOW YOUR EMOTIONS

The emotion wheel, from inner ring to outer rings:

Happy → Optimistic (Inspired, Hopeful) → Peaceful (Thankful, Sensitive) → Trusting (Intimate, Loving) → Powerful → Accepted → Proud → Interested → Content → Let down → Humiliated → Bitter → Aggressive → Frustrated → Critical

Inner ring segments: Happy, Fearful, Disgusted, Sad, Bad, Surprised, Angry

Happy outer labels: Inspired, Sensitive, Intimate, Thankful, Loving, Creative, Courageous, Valued, Respected, Confident, Successful, Inquisitive, Curious, Joyful, Free, Hopeful

Fearful outer labels: Helpless, Frightened, Worried, Inadequate, Insecure, Anxious, Scared, Rejected, Threatened

Disgusted outer labels: Persecuted, Worthless, Insignificant, Excluded, Nervous, Exposed, Judgemental, Appalled, Revolted, Nauseated, Horrified, Hesitant, Disapproving, Awful, Repelled

Sad outer labels: Hurt, Disappointed, Inferior, Empty, Remorseful, Ashamed, Powerless, Grief, Fragile, Victimized, Abandoned, Isolated, Lonely, Vulnerable, Despair, Guilty, Depressed, Hurt

Bad outer labels: Tired, Sleepy, Unfocused, Out of control, Overwhelmed, Rushed, Pressured, Apathetic, Indifferent, Busy, Stressed, Bored

Surprised outer labels: Shocked, Awe, Eager, Energetic, Dismayed, Disillusioned, Perplexed, Astonished, Startled, Confused, Amazed, Excited

Angry outer labels: Jealous, Ridiculed, Betrayed, Dismissive, Numb, Withdrawn, Annoyed, Hostile, Furious, Indignant, Disrespected, Resentful, Let down, Humiliated, Bitter, Aggressive, Frustrated, Critical

1. Which 3 emotions best describe how movement makes you feel currently?

_____

_____

_____

_____

_____

2. Which 3 emotions are most difficult for you to feel in general?

_____

_____

_____

_____

_____

_____

3. Choose 3 emotions and describe how they feel physically in your body?

_____

_____

_____

_____

_____

_____

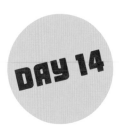

DAY 14

WHAT MOVEMENT MAKES YOU FEEL GOOD?

Choose an activity from the list you created on Day 9 to try (see page 43). Once you have tried the activity, answer the questions below to reflect on whether it was the right or wrong type of movement for you.

Name of activity: _____

Duration of activity: _____

Intensity:　0　1　2　3　4　5　6　7　8　9　10

Low   High

How did you feel before?

_____

_____

How did you feel during?

_____

_____

How did you feel after?

_____

_____

Highlight of activity?

_____

_____

Lowlight of activity?

_____

_____

Rating out of 10:

_____

Notes

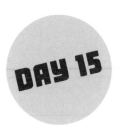

FITNESS COMES IN ALL SHAPES AND SIZES

Challenge your assumptions by learning more about everyday athletes who come in all shapes and sizes. Diversify who you are getting your motivation and inspiration from by researching four new movement heroes. Find a photo and create a profile about them.

Stick a photo here

Name: _____ Activity: _____

A bit about them: _____

_____

_____

Why they inspire me: _____

_____

_____

Stick a photo here

Name: _____ Activity: _____

A bit about them: _____

_____

_____

Why they inspire me: _____

_____

_____

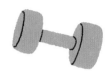

Stick a photo here

Name: _____ Activity: _____

A bit about them: _____

_____

_____

Why they inspire me: _____

_____

_____

Stick a photo here

Name: _____ Activity: _____

A bit about them: _____

_____

_____

Why they inspire me: _____

_____

_____

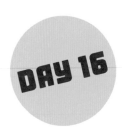

DAY 16

BENEFITS OF REGULAR MOVEMENT

Reminding yourself of the benefits of movement can help fill your motivation cup so that on the occasions when your motivation is low, you can remember why you choose to move.

Note all the ways you benefit from exercise here.

My physical benefits

- _____
  _____
- _____
  _____
- _____
  _____
- _____
  _____
- _____
  _____
- _____
  _____
- _____
  _____
- _____
  _____

My emotional benefits

- _____
  _____

- _____
  _____

- _____
  _____

- _____
  _____

- _____
  _____

- _____
  _____

- _____
  _____

- _____
  _____

Complete these sentences:

Movement makes me feel... _____
_____

Exercise helps me to... _____
_____

I wish I'd known that exercise is _____ when I was younger.

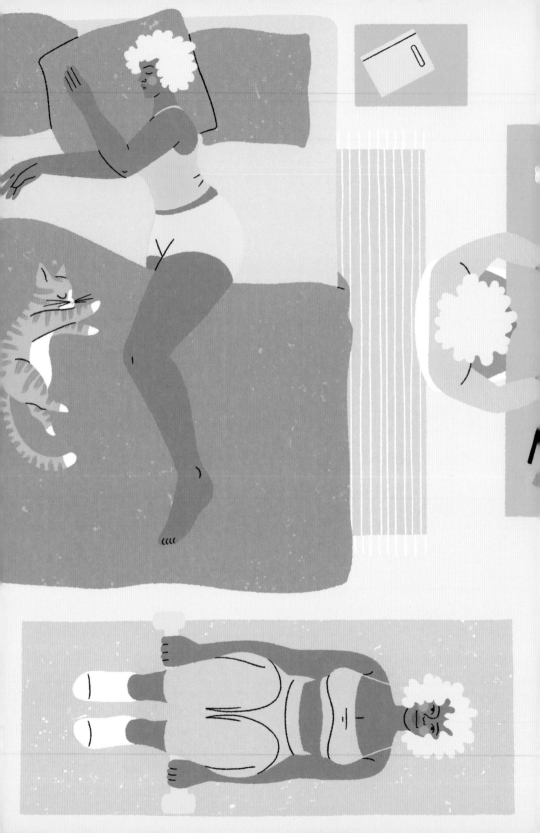

"

Now when I train, it's because it makes my head feel good, not because it might change my body shape.

– JADE

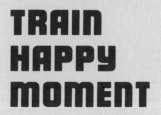

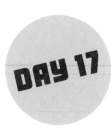

DAY 17

CREATING MORE BRAIN SPACE

Diet culture takes up a lot of our time, energy and valuable brain space. Let's reclaim it by reflecting on what you would prefer to be spending your time, money and mental energy focusing on.

Add your own examples to both the Diet Culture brain and the Intuitive Movement brain.

CALORIE COUNTING

FOOD FEAR

GUILT

DIET BOOKS

DIET CULTURE

SCALES

STEPS

BODY SHAME

EARN & BURN

TRACKING FOOD

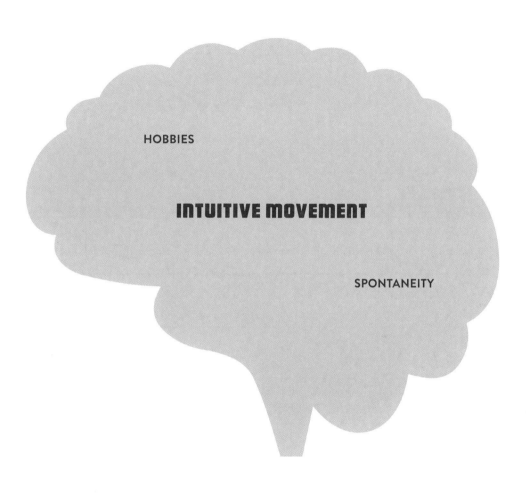

HOBBIES

INTUITIVE MOVEMENT

SPONTANEITY

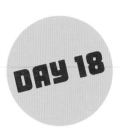

DAY 18

DECONSTRUCTING YOUR WORKOUT RULES

Choose another workout rule from Day 3 (see page 30) and deconstruct it by answering these questions.

What's the rule?

_____

_____

Where did the rule come from?

_____

_____

How do you feel if you don't stick to this rule?

_____

_____

_____

_____

_____

How could you challenge this rule and break it in the future?

_____

_____

_____

_____

_____

Notes

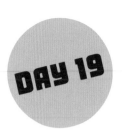

DAY 19

REST DAY CHECK-IN

It's time to reflect on how you feel about rest, and the idea of unconditional permission to rest.

How did you spend your most recent rest day?

_____

_____

_____

_____

_____

_____

_____

_____

What did you learn about your mind and body from taking a rest day?

_____

_____

_____

_____

_____

_____

_____

_____

_____

_____

What's the easiest thing about rest days?

_____

_____

_____

_____

_____

_____

What's the hardest thing about rest days?

_____

_____

_____

_____

_____

In what other ways have you been honouring your body's need for rest besides taking rest days? (For example, reaching out to a friend.)

_____

_____

_____

_____

_____

_____

_____

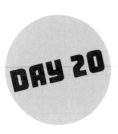

LEARNING TO LISTEN TO YOUR BODY

You may not know the answer right away, but take the time to listen to your body and understand its different cues.

Fill in each section with the obvious and subtle ways your body communicates with you.

Energy feels like:

_____

_____

_____

_____

Exhaustion feels like:

_____

_____

_____

_____

Fatigue feels like:

_____

_____

_____

_____

Comfortable effort feels like:

_____

_____

_____

_____

_____

_____

Moderate effort feels like:

_____

_____

_____

_____

_____

_____

Hard effort feels like:

_____

_____

_____

_____

_____

_____

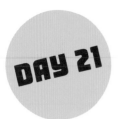

DAY 21

WHAT MOVEMENT MAKES YOU FEEL GOOD?

Pick a new activity from the list you created on Day 9 (see page 43). Give it a go and answer these questions once you have tried it.

Name of activity: _____

Duration of activity: _____

Intensity: | 0 | 1 | 2 | 3 | 4 | 5 | 6 | 7 | 8 | 9 | 10 |

Low   High

How did you feel before?
_____
_____

How did you feel during?
_____
_____

How did you feel after?
_____
_____

Highlight of activity?
_____
_____

Lowlight of activity?
_____
_____

Rating out of 10:
_____

Notes

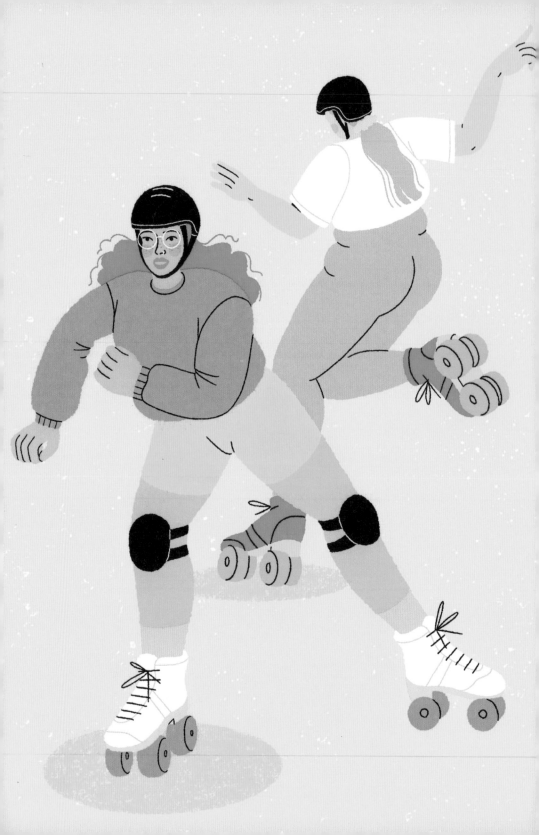

"

I started to realize that swimming was giving me some calm and I found myself visiting the pool a couple of times a week. A year later I plucked up the courage to attend adult swimming lessons and learnt the once feared front crawl. I now feel empowered from learning this new skill. Front crawling up and down the lanes brings me a joy I hadn't known before.

– REBECCA B

TRAIN HAPPY MOMENT

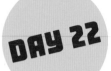

MOTIVATION TO MOVE!

Diet culture keeps us focused on the external rewards of exercise by making it all about gaining validation for our appearance.

To cultivate a deeper and more sustainable sense of motivation, we need to explore the reasons you enjoy and benefit from movement that are intrinsic to you, so you no longer need to rely on external factors to get you motivated.

Start by thinking about all the extrinsic reasons you may have used for motivation in the past. Then work on building up the list of intrinsic reasons for lasting motivation.

Start the list today and add more reasons as and when you experience them.

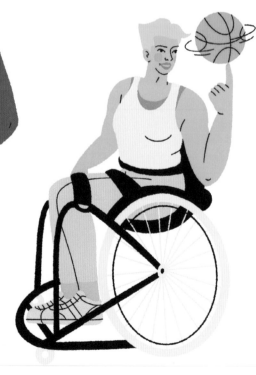

Extrinsic Reasons	Intrinsic Reasons
Example: To look good for a holiday.	*Example: To feel good.*

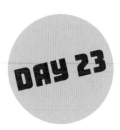

DAY 23

FOCUS ON WHAT YOUR BODY CAN DO

Let's celebrate and appreciate what your body can do in the context of fitness and in your life beyond workouts too.

Write around the body all the great things it is capable of – I've given you a few examples.

MY BODY CAN...

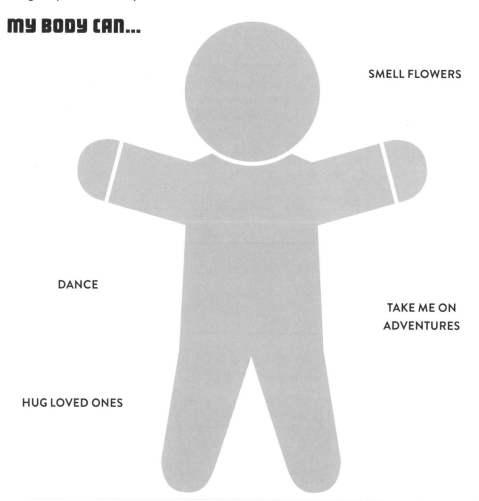

SMELL FLOWERS

DANCE

TAKE ME ON ADVENTURES

HUG LOVED ONES

Notes

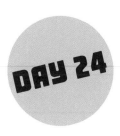

DAY 24

ALL MOVEMENT IS EQUAL

Did you used to think there were 'good' types of movement and 'bad' types of movement? Well, as a way to challenge this and neutralize the way we think about movement, it's important to acknowledge the preconceptions you may have had.

Let's reflect on what those may have been and why you thought that way by filling in these tables.

What exercise did you consider 'bad'?	Why did you think that?

What exercise did you consider 'good'?	Why did you think that?

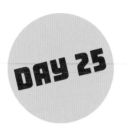

BUILD YOUR BEST WORKOUT ENVIRONMENT

DAY 25

Have you ever thought about the workout environment that's best for you? Here's your chance to reflect on and select your preferences. Answer the questions and circle your choices.

Favourite time to work out?

Early Morning   Morning   Lunchtime   Afternoon   Evening

Favourite workout outfit to wear?

_____

Music?   Yes   No

Location?   Indoors   Outdoors

Do you prefer?   Group setting   Individual

Do you prefer?   Following an instructor or plan   Doing your own thing

How long?   10 mins & under   30 mins & under   45 mins & under   1hr & under

Anything to add?

_____

_____

_____

_____

_____

_____

_____

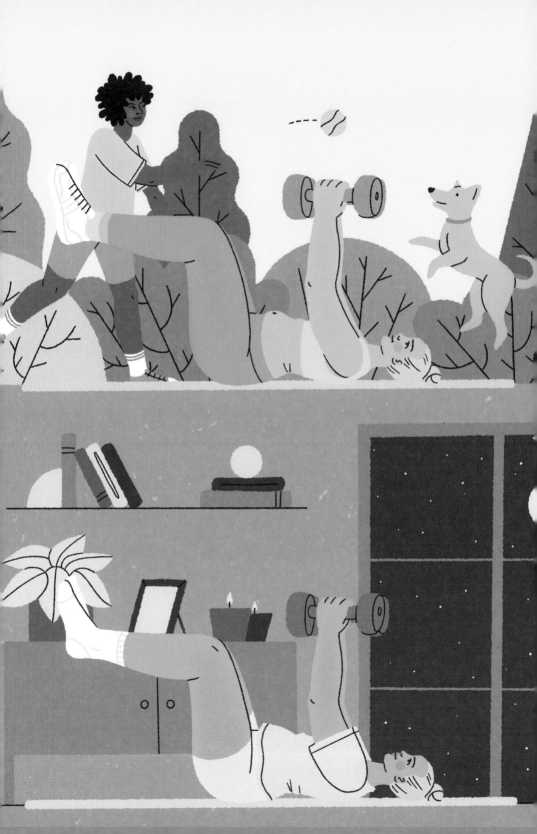

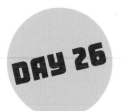

DAY 26

FITNESS TRACKER CHECK-IN

On a scale from 0–10, how easy has it been to stop tracking your workouts?

| 0 | 1 | 2 | 3 | 4 | 5 | 6 | 7 | 8 | 9 | 10 |

Easy   Moderate   Really Hard

Have you felt a difference between how movement feels when you do and don't track?

Movement when I track VS Movement without tracking

NUMBERS
DON'T
DEFINE
YOUR
WORKOUT

"

The message that exercise should be fun and make you feel good has finally sunk in, and those two things have become my goal for each session rather than closing out the rings on my watch.

– AILSA

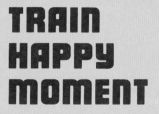

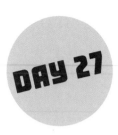

DAY 27

DECONSTRUCTING YOUR WORKOUT RULES

Once again, we are reflecting on the workout rules from Day 3 (see page 30). Choose one and deconstruct it by answering the questions.

What's the rule?

_____

_____

Where did the rule come from?

_____

_____

How can you break it?

_____

_____

_____

_____

_____

How did it feel to challenge the rule?

_____

_____

_____

_____

_____

Notes

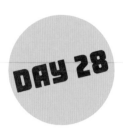

DAY 28

CELEBRATING THE VICTORIES!

We often get bogged down by focusing on the difficult or negative part of our workouts. Instead, I challenge you to start collecting and celebrating all the mini workout wins you have had to celebrate your progress!

MY WORKOUT WINS...

_____
_____
_____

_____
_____
_____

_____
_____
_____

_____
_____
_____

_____
_____
_____

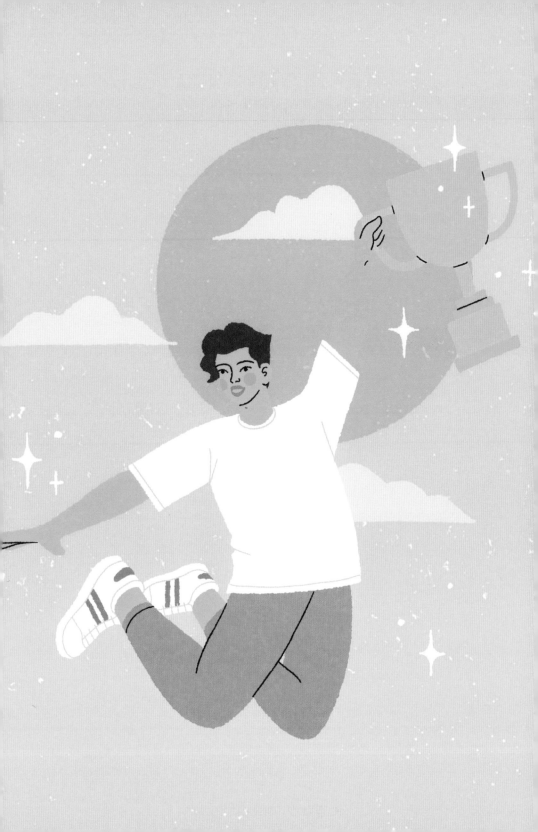

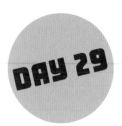

TRACKING FITNESS PROGRESS

Write down the ways that you used to track progress when following the rules of diet culture.

_____

_____

_____

_____

_____

_____

_____

_____

_____

_____

_____

_____

_____

An intuitive movement approach encourages you to shift away from tracking what you look like and how many calories you burn. Instead, focus on improving how you feel about movement as well as on what you are able to do! Use the tables on pages 89 and 90 as templates to help you get started.

Side note: only reintroduce tracking if and when you feel ready. That may well be long after this initial 30-Day Challenge.

MOOD TRACKER

Activity/Exercise	How do I feel before	How do I feel during	How do I feel after	Notes

WORKOUT TRACKER – RESISTANCE

Activity/Exercise	Week 1: Weight & reps	Week 4: Weight & reps	Week 8: Weight & reps	Week 12: Weight & reps

OR YOU CAN TRY:

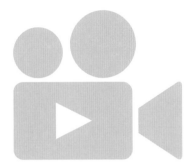

- Taking video progress of a skill/exercise. For example, record a dance routine to see if you have improved.

- Doing a fitness test regularly. For example, running a mile. Track your pace and comfort.

A REMINDER: it is not an obligation to track progress – just moving for the sake of moving is wonderful too! There is no pressure to set goals if you don't want to at this time or ever.

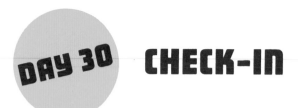

DAY 30 CHECK-IN

MY INTUITIVE MOVEMENT MOOD METER

Circle the numbers below to reflect how you feel about movement now.

How do you feel about movement?

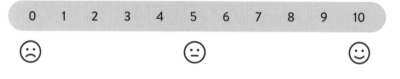

| 0 | 1 | 2 | 3 | 4 | 5 | 6 | 7 | 8 | 9 | 10 |

How motivated to move do you feel?

| 0 | 1 | 2 | 3 | 4 | 5 | 6 | 7 | 8 | 9 | 10 |

How do you feel about your body image?

| 0 | 1 | 2 | 3 | 4 | 5 | 6 | 7 | 8 | 9 | 10 |

How do you feel about your mental wellbeing?

| 0 | 1 | 2 | 3 | 4 | 5 | 6 | 7 | 8 | 9 | 10 |

What are your 3 biggest takeaways from the past 30 days?

_____

_____

_____

_____

_____

_____

_____

What has been the biggest challenge?

_____

_____

_____

_____

_____

What do you want to continue to work on?

_____

_____

_____

_____

_____

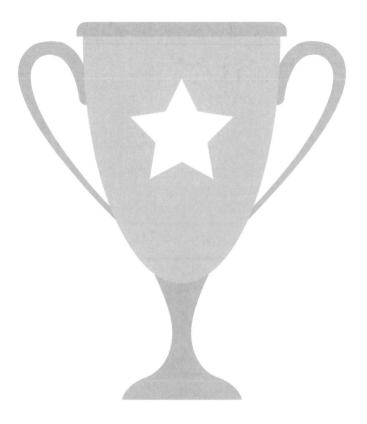

WELL DONE FOR GETTING THIS FAR!

Congratulations on doing the hard, inner work and completing the 30-Day Challenge! The tasks aren't always easy, but I hope this time of reflection has helped guide you on your path to a more positive and peaceful relationship with movement and your body.

This likely isn't the end, but just the beginning of your intuitive movement journey. Keep going!

TRAIN HAPPY MOMENTS

What does it mean to Train Happy? Well, here is how I define it:

*To move your body on your own terms in a way that feels good,
brings joy and comes from a place of care and respect.*

WHAT IS A TRAIN HAPPY MOMENT?

1. An experience of moving or resting your body on your own terms and feeling a sense of trust and connection when doing so.
2. Celebrating a win against diet culture.

Bearing all this in mind, as well as including a selection of real-life examples I also wanted to include a section for you to record your own Train Happy Moments, during and long after the 30-Day Challenge.

These moments should celebrate your wins and remind you of how far you've come – and keep you motivated and inspired to continue challenging the old beliefs and behaviours that no longer serve you. You might have a Train Happy Moment when you least expect. Using this journal to document them will serve as a reminder to keep going.

Use the templates on the following pages to record your Train Happy Moments.

MY TRAIN HAPPY MOMENT...

_____
_____
_____
_____
_____
_____
_____
_____
_____

MY TRAIN HAPPY MOMENT...

_____
_____
_____
_____
_____
_____
_____
_____
_____

MY TRAIN HAPPY MOMENT...

_____
_____
_____
_____
_____
_____
_____
_____
_____
_____

MY TRAIN HAPPY MOMENT...

_____
_____
_____
_____
_____
_____
_____
_____
_____
_____

MY TRAIN HAPPY MOMENT...

_____
_____
_____
_____
_____
_____
_____
_____
_____
_____

MY TRAIN HAPPY MOMENT...

_____
_____
_____
_____
_____
_____
_____
_____
_____
_____

MY TRAIN HAPPY MOMENT...

_____
_____
_____
_____
_____
_____
_____
_____
_____

MY TRAIN HAPPY MOMENT...

_____
_____
_____
_____
_____
_____
_____
_____
_____

MY TRAIN HAPPY MOMENT...

_____
_____
_____
_____
_____
_____
_____
_____
_____
_____

MY TRAIN HAPPY MOMENT...

_____
_____
_____
_____
_____
_____
_____
_____
_____
_____

MY TRAIN HAPPY MOMENT...

_____

_____

_____

_____

_____

_____

_____

_____

_____

MY TRAIN HAPPY MOMENT...

_____

_____

_____

_____

_____

_____

_____

_____

_____

MY TRAIN HAPPY MOMENT...

_____
_____
_____
_____
_____
_____
_____
_____
_____

MY TRAIN HAPPY MOMENT...

_____
_____
_____
_____
_____
_____
_____
_____
_____

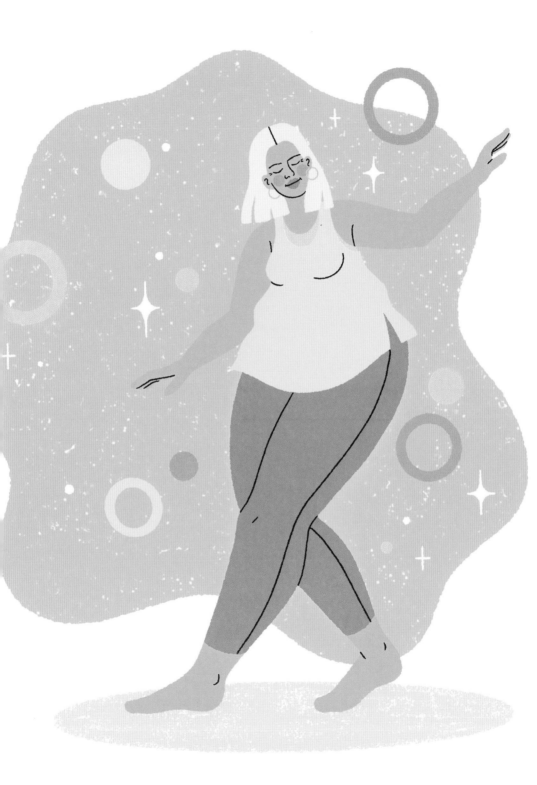

Notes

Notes

Notes

Notes

Notes

Notes

Notes

FURTHER READING

Body Respect by Linda Bacon and Lucy Aphramor
Fitness for Every Body by Meg Boggs
Health at Every Size by Linda Bacon
Intuitive Eating (4th edition) by Evelyn Tribole and Elyse Resch
More Than a Body by Lindsay Kite and Lexie Kite

MORE FROM TALLY RYE

You can learn more about my work by reading my first book, listening to my podcast and following me on social media.

READ
Train Happy: An Intuitive Exercise Plan for Every Body

LISTEN
Train Happy Podcast
www.tallyrye.co.uk/podcast

FOLLOW
Instagram, Twitter and TikTok: @tallyrye
www.tallyrye.co.uk

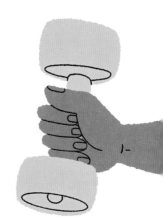

ACKNOWLEDGEMENTS

Thank you to Evelyn Tribole and Elyse Resch whose work inspired *Train Happy* and the principles of Intuitive Movement.

Thank you to Ailsa, Christal, Jade, Krista, Nicola, Rebecca B and Rebecca K, for sharing their Train Happy Moments.

A big **THANK YOU** to my online community and in-person clients for inspiring and motivating me to want to change the fitness industry for the better.

And of course thank you to my family, my partner Jack and my hugely supportive friends.

First published in the United Kingdom in 2021 by
Pavilion
43 Great Ormond Street
London
WC1N 3HZ

ISBN: 9781911682257

A CIP catalogue record for this book is available from the British Library.
10 9 8 7 6 5 4 3 2 1

Reproduction by Rival Colour Ltd., UK
Printed and bound by IMAK Ofset, Turkey

www.pavilionbooks.com

Publisher's Acknowledgements
The wheel of emotion on page 52 was inspired by Geoffrey Roberts's
Emotional Word Wheel.

Commissioning Editor: Cara Armstrong
Project Editor: Krissy Mallett
Design Manager: Nicky Collings
Layout Designer: Hannah Naughton
Illustrations by Andrea Oerter
Production Controller: Phil Brown

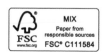